YOUR KNOWLEDGE HAS VALUE

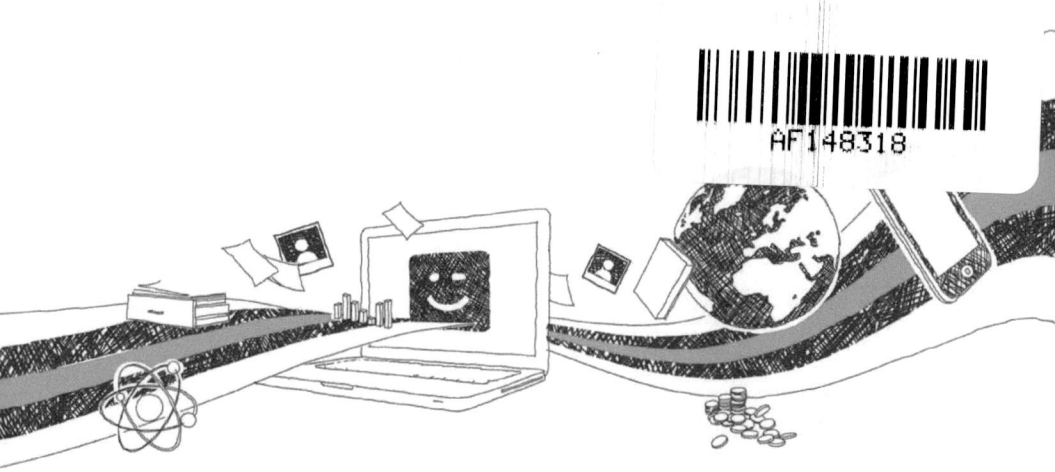
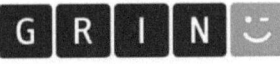

Bibliographic information published by the German National Library:

The German National Library lists this publication in the National Bibliography; detailed bibliographic data are available on the Internet at http://dnb.dnb.de .

Imprint:

Copyright © 2008 GRIN Verlag, Open Publishing GmbH
Print and binding: Books on Demand GmbH, Norderstedt Germany
ISBN: 9783668285460

This book at GRIN:

http://www.grin.com/en/e-book/338391/apoliprotein-b-a1-and-diabetes-type-2

Reaz Mazumdar

Apoliprotein B, A1 and Diabetes Type 2

GRIN Publishing

GRIN - Your knowledge has value

Since its foundation in 1998, GRIN has specialized in publishing academic texts by students, college teachers and other academics as e-book and printed book. The website www.grin.com is an ideal platform for presenting term papers, final papers, scientific essays, dissertations and specialist books.

Visit us on the internet:

http://www.grin.com/

http://www.facebook.com/grincom

http://www.twitter.com/grin_com

Contents

Apoliprotein B, A1 and Diabetes Type 2

Reaz Mohammad Mazumdar
BCSIR, Dhaka, Bangladesh

Diabetes mellitus refers to a group of metabolic disorders of multiple aetiology and characterized by chronic hyperglycaemia with disturbances of carbohydrate, fat and protein metabolism resulting from defects in insulin secretion, insulin action, or both. The effects of diabetes mellitus include long–term damage, dysfunction and failure of various organs. Diabetes mellitus may present with characteristic symptoms such as thirst, polyuria, blurring of vision, and weight loss. In its most severe forms, ketoacidosis or a non–ketotic hyperosmolar state may develop and lead to stupor, coma and in absence of effective treatment, death. Often symptoms are not severe, or may be absent, and consequently hyperglycaemia sufficient to cause pathological and functional changes may be present for a long time before the diagnosis is made (WHO, 1999). It is a major health problem in all nations. Diabetes is the single, most important metabolic disease, widely recognized as one of the leading causes of death and disability worldwide (Zimmet, 1999; Songer, 1995). This devastating disease can affect nearly every system in the body. It can cause blindness, lead to end stage renal disease, lower extremity amputations and increase the risk for stroke, ischemic heart disease, peripheral vascular disease, and neuropathy. Diabetic macro and microvascular complications are resulting in increased disability and enormous health care costs (IDF, 2003).

The Global prevalence of diabetes for all age-groups was estimated to be 2.8% in 2000 and 4.4% in 2030 (Wild *et al.,* 2004). Total number of people with diabetes is projected to rise from 171 million in 2000 to 366 million in 2030. Overall, diabetes prevalence is higher in men, but there are more women with diabetes than men (Scrichard *et al.*, 2004). The largest proportional and absolute increase will occur in developing countries, where the prevalence will rise from 4.2 to 5.6%, and in Bangladesh, from 3.9 to 4.8%. In developing countries, the majority of people with diabetes are in the 45 to 64 years age range. In the European Region, an average total diabetes prevalence of 7.8 % in the adult population (20 - 79 years) or 48.4 million persons has been estimated in 2003 (IDF, 2003). Without effective prevention programs, diabetes prevalence in Europe is expected to increase to 9.1 % or 58.6 millions in 2025 as estimated by the International Diabetes Federation (IDF, 2003). Number of community based studies conducted in Bangladesh at different time points have revealed an increasing trend of diabetes prevalence ranging from 1.5 to 3.8% in the semi-urban and

2

rural communities (West *et al.,* 1966; Mahtab *et al.,* 1983; Sayeed *et al.,* 1995; Sayeed *et al.,* 1997). In a recent study the prevalence of diabetic patients in Bangladeshi urban population was found to be 7.97% and age adjusted prevalence of diabetes found to be higher in urban than the rural population subjects (Sayeed *et al.,* 1997).

Classification of Diabetes

According to the present classification of diabetes four main classes of the disease are type 1, type 2, Other Specific Types and Gestational Diabetes Mellitus (Table 1) (WHO, 1999 and ADA, 1997). Impaired glucose tolerance (IGT) was an allied category of glucose intolerance in the WHO technical report (1985) but absent in the new classification by WHO (1999). The class "Impaired Glucose Tolerance" is now classified as a stage of impaired glucose regulation, since it can be observed in any hyperglycaemic disorder, and is itself not diabetes. A clinical stage of Impaired Fasting Glycaemia (IFG) has been introduced to classify individuals who have fasting glucose values above the normal range, but below those diagnostic of diabetes (WHO, 1999). Together they are termed as prediabetes.

Table 1: Aetiological Classification of Disorders of Glycaemia (WHO, 1999)

Type 1 (beta-cell destruction, usually leading to absolute insulin deficiency)
Autoimmune
Idiopathic
Type 2 (may range from predominantly insulin resistance with relative insulin deficiency to a predominantly secretory defect with or without insulin resistance)
Other specific types
Genetic defects of beta-cell function
Genetic defects in insulin action
Diseases of the exocrine pancreas
Endocrinopathies
Drug- or chemical-induced
Infections
Uncommon forms of immune-mediated diabetes
Other genetic syndromes sometimes associated with diabetes
Gestational diabetes

Type 1 diabetes mellitus

Type 1 diabetes (T1DM) is thought to be caused by autoimmune-mediated destruction of pancreatic β-cell islets, resulting in near absolute insulin deficiency (Harris, 2000). T1DM is characterized by sudden onset of symptoms, proneness to ketoacidosis and need of insulin for survival. The hallmark of the T1DM is pancreatic B cell damage resulting in very low to absolute loss of insulin secretion. T1DM mainly seen in children and young adults and accounts for about 10% of all diabetic patients (ADA, 1997). T1DM is divided on the basis of type of damage of B cells; immune mediated type 1 (Type 1A) and non-immune mediated type 1 (idiopathic type 1, T1B) (ADA, 1997; WHO, 1999). The exact etiological factor(s) are still unknown; multiple genetic and environmental factors are thought to be involved (ADA, 1997; WHO, 1999).

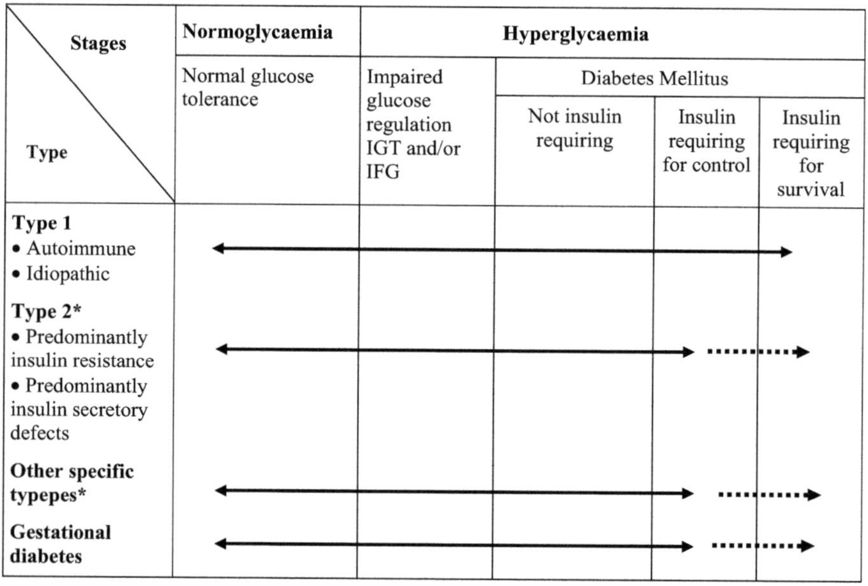

Stages / Type	Normoglycaemia	Hyperglycaemia			
	Normal glucose tolerance	Impaired glucose regulation IGT and/or IFG	Diabetes Mellitus		
			Not insulin requiring	Insulin requiring for control	Insulin requiring for survival
Type 1 • Autoimmune • Idiopathic	←				→
Type 2* • Predominantly insulin resistance • Predominantly insulin secretory defects	←			······→	
Other specific typepes*	←			·····→	
Gestational diabetes	←			·····→	

* In rare instances patients in these categories (eg Vacor Toxicity, Type 1 presenting in pregnancy, etc) may require insulin for survival.

Figure 1: Disorders of Glycemia: aetiological types and clinical stages (WHO, 1999).

Type 2 Diabetes Mellitus

Type 2 diabetes mellitus (T2DM) accounts for over 90% of cases globally. T2DM is characterized by insulin resistance and/or abnormal insulin secretion, either of which may predominate. People with type 2 diabetes are not dependent on exogenous insulin, but may require it for control of blood glucose levels if this is not achieved with diet alone or with oral hypoglycaemic agents (GCDE) and constitutes 90- 95% of cases (Harris, 2000; Bergenstal *et al.*, 2001).

Gestational Diabetes

Gestational diabetes is carbohydrate intolerance resulting in hyperglycaemia of variable severity with onset or first recognition during pregnancy. Gestational diabetes affects 3-5% of all.

Other specific types

Other specific types are less common forms of diabetes mellitus, but there are those in which the underlying defect or disease processes can be identified in a relatively specific manner. They include, for example, fibrocalculous pancreatopathy, a form of diabetes, which was formerly classified as one type of malnutrition-related diabetes mellitus (ADA, 2005).

Prediabetes

Impaired glucose regulation (IGR) or "Prediabetes" is the term used to describe the condition in which blood glucose levels are higher than normal but yet not diabetic. Subjects with impaired fasting glucose (IFG) and/or impaired glucose tolerance (IGT) are referred to as IGR or Prediabetes. The term "Impaired glucose regulation" (IGR) was used by World Health Organization (WHO) and "Prediabetes" by American Diabetic Association (ADA). IGR refers to a metabolic state between normal glucose homeostasis and diabetes. They are not interchangeable and represent different abnormalities of glucose regulation, one in fasting state and one postprandial (WHO, 1999). According to fasting and post load glucose concentration, at present patients with IGR or prediabetes may be stratified into (i) Isolated Impaired glucose tolerance (IGT); (ii) Isolated Impaired fasting glucose (IFG) and; (iII) Combined IFG-IGT (WHO and ADA, 2002).

Impaired glucose tolerance

Impaired glucose tolerance (IGT) is defined as fasting plasma glucose <6.1mmol/l and 2h plasma glucose between 7.8 and 11.0 mmol/l (ADA, 2005). Historically the term IGT was first introduced by the National Diabetes Data Group in 1979 and later, the same word was endorsed by WHO in 1980. In the adult population, age range 20-79 yrs, prevalence of IGT is projected to increase globally from 8.2 in the year 2003 to 9.0% in 2025 and in the same period in Bangladesh from 7.1 to 7.8% (Sicree *et al.*, 2003). IGT is found to be more prevalent than IFG. The prevalence of IGT rises in old age (Unwin *et al., 2002*). The age standard prevalence of IFG in European population found to be round 11.8 % (Boronat *et al.*, 2002). In a study involving Dutch population the prevalence of IGT was shown to be 13.8 % in men and 14.6% in women (Corpeleijn *et al.*, 2006). IGT patients were followed up for 11 years in Mauritius and of them 46% found to develop diabetes, 28% remained unchanged in category, 4% developed IFG, and glucose levels normalized in 24%. A study by Shaw et al (1999) followed up adult IFG cases and of them 38% developed diabetes, 7% remained unchanged, 17% developed IGT and 38% achieved normal glucose.

Impaired fasting glucose

Impaired fasting glucose (IFG) is defined as fasting plasma glucose between 6.1 and 6.9 mmol/l and 2h plasma glucose <7.8 mmol/l (ADA, 2005). In 1997, the ADA published report mentioned IFG as a new category, which was also adopted in 1999 World Health Organization (WHO) report (Stern and Burke, 2000). Recently American Diabetic Association (ADA) has reduced the lower cut off value of fasting plasma glucose in IFG from 6.1 mmol/l to 5.6 mmol/l (ADA, 2005). IFG found to be more common among men. The prevalence of IFG tends to plateau in middle age (Unwin *et al., 2002*). The crude prevalence of IFG was found to be 12.4% in rural population of Bangladesh and age-standardized prevalence, however, was 13.0% (Sayeed *et al.,* 2003). Prevalence of IFG among Dutch population found to be 9.7% in men and 6.1% in women (Corpeleijn *et al.*, 2005). However, age standard prevalence of IFG in European population was earlier shown to be 2.8% (Boronat *et al.,* 2002).

Combined IFG-IGT

A reasonable number of subjects, both in abroad and in Bangladesh found to have blood glucose level at the range of IFG and IGT and they are frequently known as IFG-IGT subjects; subjects with fasting plasma glucose between 6.1mmol/l and 6.9 mmol/l and 2h plasma glucose between 7.8mmol/l and 11.0 mmol/l (ADA, 2005). A group of combined IFG-IGT subjects were followed up and progression of this combined IFG-IGT to diabetes was found to be 28% per year (Rasmussen *et al.*, 2007).

Feature of IFG/ IGT

The main feature of IFG and/ or IGT are: 1) a stage in the natural history of disordered glucose metabolism, 2) can lead to any type of diabetes, 3) increased risk of progression to diabetes, 4) increased risk of cardiovascular diseases 5) little or no risk of microvascular diseases, and 6) some patient may revert to normoglycemic (Balkau and Eschwege, 2003). IFG and IGT are asymptomatic and unassociated with any manifested morbidity, but their sole significance lies in the fact that they predict future diabetes or cardiovascular diseases (Stern and Burke 2000). Both IFG and IGT are similarly associated with an increased risk of diabetes mellitus. Risk is higher where IGT and IFG coexists (Unwin *et al.*, *2002*). IGT is more prevalent than IFG, less than or equal to 50% of people with IFG has IGT and 20-30% with IGT also has IFG (Unwin *et al.*, *2002*). From Diabetes Epidemiology: Collaborative analysis of Diagnostic criteria in Asia study it was found that IGT was more prevalent than IFG in all Asian peoples studied for all age groups (DECODA, 2003).

Pathophysiology of Prediabetes

Consensus Statement regarding IGT/IFG by the International Diabetes Federation (IDF) stated that 'raised hepatic glucose output and a defect in early insulin secretion are the characteristic of IFG and peripheral insulin resistance is most characteristic of IGT' (Unwin *et al.*, *2002*). This notion was supported by findings of the number of studies which have shown IFG is associated with more B cell failure (Weyer *et al.*, 1999; Davies *et al.*, 2000; Schianca *et al.*, 2003; Li *et al.*, 2003) and IGT with predominantly insulin resistance (Davies *et al.*, 2000; Schianca *et al.*, 2003; Festa *et al.*, 2004). Few have, however, shown that both IFG and IGT have similar impairment of insulin action (Weyer *et al.*, 1999; Li *et al.*, 2003). However in contrast some have claimed that subjects with IFG had more insulin resistance and features of insulin resistance and those with IGT more defective insulin secretion in early and late phase (Tripathy *et al.*, 2000; Hanefeld *et al.*, 2003). The basis for this kind of variation is still unclear. Since genetic factors are involved in both β-cell failure and insulin resistance, racial variation is expected.

A recent study involving Bangladeshi IGR subjects has shown to have different pathophysiological mechanisms in IFG, IGT and IFG-IGT subjects (Rahman *et al*, 2006). The primary defect in IFG found to be B cell dysfunction with a tendency to insulin resistance and that in IGT insulin resistantce. Combined defects are seen in IFG-IGT subjects. Difference in pathophysiology of IFG, IGT and IFG-IGT in Bangladeshi prediabetes subjects attributed to the genetic background and environmental factor(s).

Natural history of type 2 diabetes

The natural history of type 2 diabetes, starting with normal glucose tolerance, insulin resistance, and compensatory hyperinsulinemia with progression to impaired glucose tolerance (IGT) and overt diabetes mellitus has been studied in different populations; Caucasians, Native-Americans, Mexican Americans, and Pacific Islanders (Saad *et al.*, 1989; Haffner *et al.*, 1995; Weyer *et al.*, 2000; Kahn 2001; Bergman *et al.*, 2002). Type 2 diabetes was invariably associated with the presence of obesity and the close association of diabetes and obesity often termed as diabosity. The progression from normal to impaired glucose tolerance is associated with a marked increase in both fasting and glucose-stimulated plasma insulin levels (DeFronzo, 1988; Saad *et al.*, 1989; Lillioja *et al.*, 1988; Jallut *et al.*, 1990) and a decrease in tissue sensitivity to insulin. The metabolic sequences that eventually lead to T2DM precede the development of hyperglycemia by years or even decades. Insulin resistance, ie., resistance to action of insulin role in promoting glucose uptake by skeletal muscle and fat cells, is the initial metabolic defect. At first, the pancreatic β-cell is able to compensate by increasing insulin levels, leading to hyperinsulinemia. This compensation is able to keep glucose levels normalized for a period of time (up to several years), but IGT develops with mild postprandial hyperglycemia. Clinically, IFG and IGT represent a similar point along the continuum between normal glucose tolerance and frank diabetes: an essentially asymptomatic but still potentially pathological stage characterized by mild hyperglycemia. Both IGT and IFG serve as markers for those who are at greatest risk for developing T2DM. Number of clinical studies have determined the cumulative risk of developing T2DM once IGT is recognized (Rewers and Hamman, 1995). Two additional pathophysiological changes become manifest during the transition from IGT to T2DM.

8

Insulin resistance becomes more severe, a progression that may be due not only to full expression of genetic defects, but also to acquired factors such as obesity, decreased physical activity, and aging. The second change is an increase in basal hepatic glucose production. Some controversy still exists as to whether insulin resistance or inadequate insulin secretion occurs first in the pathogenesis of diabetes. However, a general consensus has emerged that insulin resistance is the primary defect in T2DM (Eriksson *et al.*, 1989).

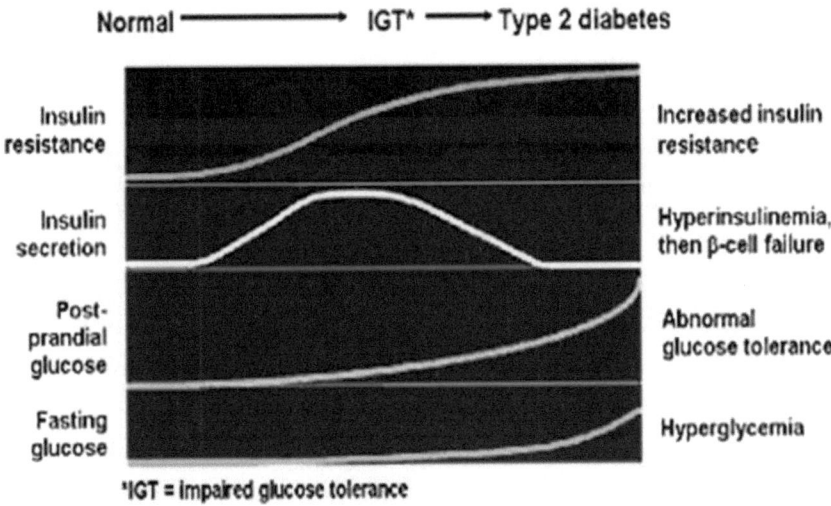

Figure 2: Insulin resistance and β-cell dysfunction combine to cause type 2 diabetes

Even though the plasma insulin response is increased two- to threefold above that in normal-glucose-tolerant subjects, overt diabetes does not develop unless a concomitant defect in insulin secretion is present. The defect in insulin secretion can be appreciated when ß-cell function is viewed relative to the prevailing severity of insulin resistance. The progression from IGT to type 2 diabetes with mild fasting hyperglycemia is heralded by an inability of the ß-cell to maintain its previously high rate of insulin secretion in response to a glucose challenge (Saad *et al.*, 1989; Saad *et al.*,1988) without any further or minimal deterioration in tissue sensitivity to insulin.

Table 2: Natural history of type 2 diabetes

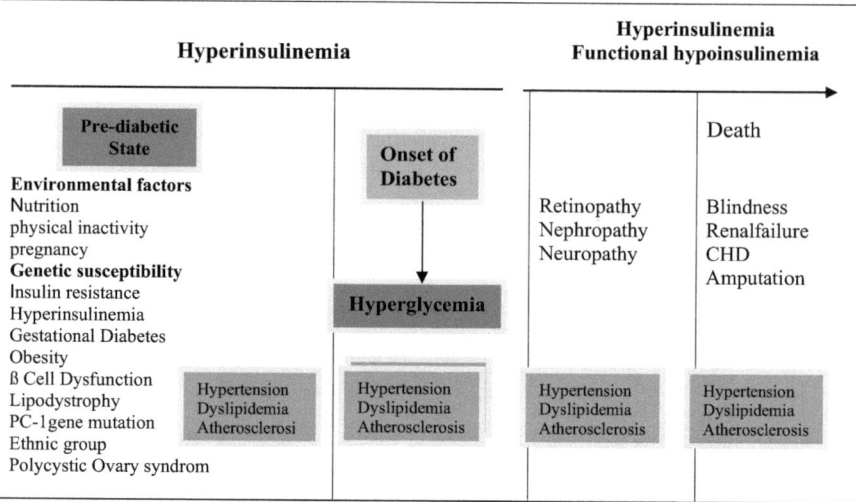

The earliest detectable abnormality that precedes the onset of diabetes mellitus is an increase in the fasting and glucose-stimulated plasma insulin concentration and a decrease in tissue sensitivity to insulin (Hansen and Bodkin, 1986). With time, this high rate of insulin secretion cannot be maintained and the downward slope of Starling's curve commences. At this point, marked fasting hyperglycemia and glucose intolerance ensue. Studies have demonstrated that hyperinsulinemia precedes the development of type 2 diabetes and hyperinsulinemia is a strong predictor of the development of IGT and type 2 diabetes (Jensen *et al.*, 2002; Dowse *et al.*, 1996; Haffner *et al.*, 1986; Ho *et al.*, 1990). A sensitive and dynamic balance between tissue sensitivity to insulin and the prevailing insulin concentration exists (Warram *et al,* 1990; Vaag *et al,* 1992). In general, type 2 diabetes develops when pancreatic β cells fail to secrete sufficient amounts of insulin to meet the metabolic demand. An increased metabolic demand for insulin due to insulin resistance in several tissues usually precedes the development of hyperglycemia. There is thus a period of normal or near-normal glycemia in which pancreatic β cells compensate for insulin resistance by hypersecretion of insulin.

At some point, however, this period of β cell compensation is followed by β cell failure, in which the pancreas fails to secrete sufficient insulin and diabetes ensues (Anderson *et al,* 2003). The decline in insulin levels, and thus a decrease in insulin's inhibitory effects, allows for increased hepatic glucose production. β-Cell exhaustion may be genetically mediated or result from hypothesized damage to the β-cell from chronic exposure to hyperglycemia, or it may result from adverse effects of increased free fatty acids. Whatever the underlying causes and mechanisms, it is clear that the full phenotypic expression of type 2 diabetes requires both insulin resistance and β-cell dysfunction.

Clinical significance of prediabetes

Risk for diabetes

Given the natural history of prediabetes, about 3%–10% of people per year with prediabetes develop diabetes. Data are particularly well substantiated for IGT. In the Diabetes Prevention Program, (Knowler et al., 2002) with subjects who had IGT, with or without IFG, there found to be about 10% annual rate of progression to diabetes in the control group. Other studies have shown similar or somewhat lower rates of progression from IGT or IFG to diabetes (Tuomilehto et al., 2001; Pan et al., 1997). It has also been shown that combination of IFG and IGT confer a greater risk for diabetes than either category alone. Prediabetes confers about a six fold risk to develop diabetes compared to those with normal glucose tolerance. In most studies the rates of conversion from IFG and IGT to diabetes found to be almost similar, however, IGT showed greater sensitivity (Unwin et al., 2002) but less specificity (Shaw et al., 1999) than IFG in predicting risk for diabetes. Each category has a similar positive predictive value (Genuth et al., 2003). Thus, many people with prediabetes (a quarter or more) may revert long term to having normal glucose tolerance, and after a protracted follow-up, only about 50% of people with IGT or IFG will develop diabetes.

Risk for Cardiovascular disease

Prediabetic subjects have an increased risk of developing cardiovascular disease (CVD) and all-cause mortality compared to the age adjusted adults with normal glucose tolerance (Decode Study Group, 2001; Coutinho et al., 1999; Liao et al., 2001). About two- to three fold increased risk for cardiovascular events was observed in younger adults with prediabetes (Zhang et al., 2003) (Bjornholt et al., 1999). This level of risk is almost similar for cardiovascular risk among T2DM (Wood et al., 1998; Liao et al., 2001). Insulin resistance found to be associated with failure to regulate VLDL production and usually there is a raised ApoB level in the VLDL, IDL and LDL classes (Chan et al., 2004, Taskinen,

11

2003). ApolipoproteinB-100 (ApoB) is present as a single molecule in low-, intermediate- and very low-density lipoproteins (LDL, IDL and VLDL, respectively) and ApoAI is the major apolipoprotein associated with high-density lipoprotein (HDL). The ApoB and ApoAI ratio (henceforth apoB/A) has been proposed to reflect the balance between the opposing processes of arterial internalization of cholesterol and the reverse transport of cholesterol back to the liver (Walldius and Jungner, 2004 and 2005). Thus, ApoB, indicates the number of potentially atherogenic lipoprotein particles, and ApoA-I, which reflects antiatherogenic HDL particles, may indicate more accurately cardiovascular (CV) risk than LDL C and other lipids (Walldius and Jungner, 2006). A number of studies have shown that IGT and normo-glycemeic subjects have rather greater risk of developing CVD than those with IFG (Decode Study Group, 2001; Coutinho *et al.,* 1999; Liao *et al.,* 2001). This was further substantiated by the fact that even after adjusting hypertension and lipid abnormalities, other known CVD risk factors, it was IGT, but possibly not IFG, remained an independent risk factor for development of CVD (Coutinho *et al.,* 1999).

APOLIPOPROTEINS

Apolipoproteins, protein components of lipoproteins, are part of the transport systems for triacyiglycerols (triglycerides) and cholesterol in blood (Erkelens, 1989). Dietary fats are digested in the intestine and carried to the liver. Fats are also synthesized in the liver itself. Fats are stored in fat cells (adipocytes). The fatty, oily components of lipoproteins are not soluble in water. But because of their detergent-like (amphipathic) properties, apolipoproteins can dissolve them. Apolipoproteins have three major functions: (i) maintaining the stability of lipoprotein particles; (ii) acting as cofactors for enzymes that act on lipoproteins, and (iii) removing lipoproteins from circulation by receptor-mediated mechanisms.

Apolipoproteins are of four mare class; apolipoproteins A (Apo A), B (Apo B), C (Apo C) and E (Apo E). Each of the three groups A, B and C consists of two or more distinct proteins. These are for ApoA: ApoA-I, ApoA-II, and ApoA-IV, for ApoB: ApoB-100 and ApoB-48; and for ApoC: ApoC-I, ApoC-II and ApoC-III. ApoE includes several isoforms. Each class of lipoproteins includes a variety of apolipoproteins in differing proportions with the exception of LDL, which contains Apo B-100 as the sole apolipoprotein. ApoA-I and ApoA-II constitute approximately 90 percent of the protein moiety of HDL whereas ApoC and ApoE are present in various proportions in chylomicrons, VLDL, IDL and HDL. ApoB-

100 is present in LDL, VLDL and IDL. ApoB-48 resides only in chylomicrons and so called chylomicron remnants (Kane, 1986). Apolipoprotein synthesis in the intestine is regulated principally by the fat content of the diet. Apolipoprotein synthesis in the liver is controlled by a host of factors, including dietary composition, hormones (insulin, glucagon, thyroxin, estrogens, androgens), alcohol intake, and various drugs (statins, niacin,and fibric acids).

Apolipoprotein A1

ApoA1 is the major apo in HDL-c particles and initiates the 'reverse cholesterol transport'. ApoA1 can 'pick up' excess cholesterol from peripheral cells and transfer it back to the liver in the HDL particles. ApoA1 also manifests anti-inflammatory and antioxidant effects (Walldius and Jungner, 2004; Marcovina and Packard, 2006; Schlitt *et al.*, 2005; Shah *et al.*, 2001; Barter and Rye, 2006). ApoA1 is not contained in the potentially atherogenic ApoB-containing particles and thus ApoA1 in most cases only reflects the athero-protective part of the metabolism. ApoA1 is considered to be the 'active ingredient' in HDL. It mediates cell–lipoprotein interactions, and is essential for cholesterol uptake into the lipoprotein and for deposition of the lipid in hepatocytes via the agency of SR-B1-like receptors (Rye *et al.*, 1999, Lewis and Rader, 2005). The protein also has anti-inflammatory and anti-oxidative properties and this may contribute to its cardioprotective role as inflammation and oxidation are believed to be key processes in atherosclerosis. HDL-c particles are smaller and contain different apolipoproteins, mainly apoA1 and apoA-II. Both these apolipoproteins have properties that protect the lipids against oxidative modification. In addition, some of the other proteins transported by HDL, such as paraoxonase, have antioxidant properties.   Therefore, whereas LDL is very susceptible to oxidative modification, HDL-c is relatively resistant to it, and this is one of the reasons underlying the anti-inflammatory properties of HDL (Rye *et al.*, 1999).

Function of ApoA-1 in HDL metabolism and reverse cholesterol transport

Cholesterol that is synthesized or deposited in peripheral tissues is returned to the liver in a process referred to as reverse cholesterol transport in which high-density lipoprotein (HDL) plays a central role. HDL may be secreted by the liver or intestine in the form of nascent particles consisting of phospholipid and apolipoprotein A-I (apoA-I).   Nascent HDL interacts with peripheral cells, such as macrophages, to facilitate the removal of excess free cholesterol (FC), a process facilitated by the ATP-binding cassette protein 1 (ABC1) gene.

FC is generated in part by the hydrolysis of intracellular cholesteryl ester (CE) stores. HDL is then converted into mature CE–rich HDL as a result of the plasma cholesterol-esterifying enzyme lecithin: cholesterol acyltransferase (LCAT), which is activated by ApoA1. CE may be removed by several different pathways, including selective uptake by the liver, i.e. the removal of lipid without the uptake of HDL proteins. Selective uptake appears to be mediated by the scavenger receptor class-B, type I (SR-BI), which is expressed in the liver and has been shown to be a receptor for HDL. CE derived from HDL contributes to the hepatic–cholesterol pool used for bile acid synthesis. Cholesterol is eventually excreted from the body either as bile acid or as free cholesterol in the bile (Fielding *et al.*, 1995; Breslow *et al.*, 1995; Acton, 1996).

Secreted CMs contain apoAs, which are transferred with phospholipids into the high-density lipoprotein (HDL) fraction during lipolysis. Similar HDL particles (HDL2) may be formed as a byproduct of the lipolysis of VLDL. Hepatic lipase, found primarily on the endothelium of the hepatic sinusoids, hydrolyses HDL2 TG and phospholipids to form small HDL3 particles, which may be cleared by the kidney. Mature HDL3 and HDL2 are generated from lipid-free Apo A1 or lipid-poor pre-ß1-HDL as the precursors. These precursors are produced as nascent HDL by the liver or intestine, or are released from lipolysed VLDL and chylomicrons or released by interconversion of HDL3 and HDL2. ABC1-mediated lipid efflux from cells is important for initial lipidation; LCAT-mediated esterification of cholesterol generates spherical particles that continue to grow on ongoing cholesterol esterification and PLTP-mediated particle fusion and surface remnant transfer. Larger HDL2 particles are converted into smaller HDL3 particles on CETP-mediated export of cholesteryl esters from HDL onto: apo B-containing lipoproteins, SR-BI–mediated selective uptake of cholesteryl esters into liver and steroidogenic organs, and HL- and EL-mediated hydrolysis of phospholipids. HDL lipids are catabolized either separately from HDL proteins (ie, by selective uptake or via CETP transfer) or together with HDL proteins (i.e., via uptake through as-yet-unknown HDL receptors or apo E receptors). The conversion of HDL2 into HDL3 and the PLTP-mediated conversion of HDL3 into HDL2-liberated lipid-free or poorly lipidated apo A1. A portion of lipid-free apo A1 undergoes glomerular filtration in the kidney and tubular reabsorption through cubilin (von-Eckardstein and Assmann, 2000).

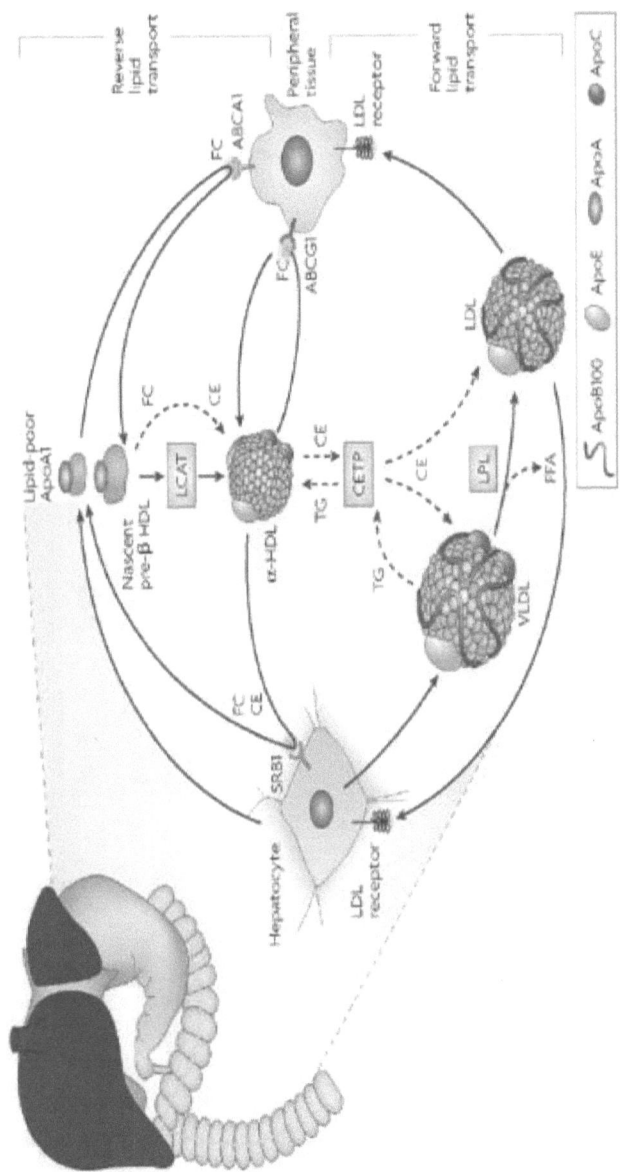

Figure 3: Lipid poor apolipoproteinA1 produced by liver and intestine.

[1] https://www.researchgate.net/publication/5768349/figure/fig3/AS:278988464377856@1443527441101/Figure-2-Lipoprotein-metabolismDuring-reverse-lipid-transport-apolipoprotein-A1.png

ApoA1 and HDL cholesterol level determining factors

The factors which determine HDL cholesterol and Apo AI levels have only recently been understood (Brewer, 2004) (Figure 4). Major influences on circulating HDL levels: (i) the efflux of cholesterol from the liver through ATP Binding Cassette AI (ABCAI). This cholesterol combining with apolipoprotein AI (apo AI) creates an HDL particle large enough to avoid glomerular filtration; (ii) the rate of removal of cholesteryl ester (CE) from HDL under the agency of CETP; and (iii) the rate of removal of CE from HDL by hepatic Scavenger Receptor B1 (SR-B1, also known as CLA-1) (Brewer, 2004). HDL undergoes constant remodeling with exchange of lipid and protein components between HDL subspecies and with other lipoproteins.

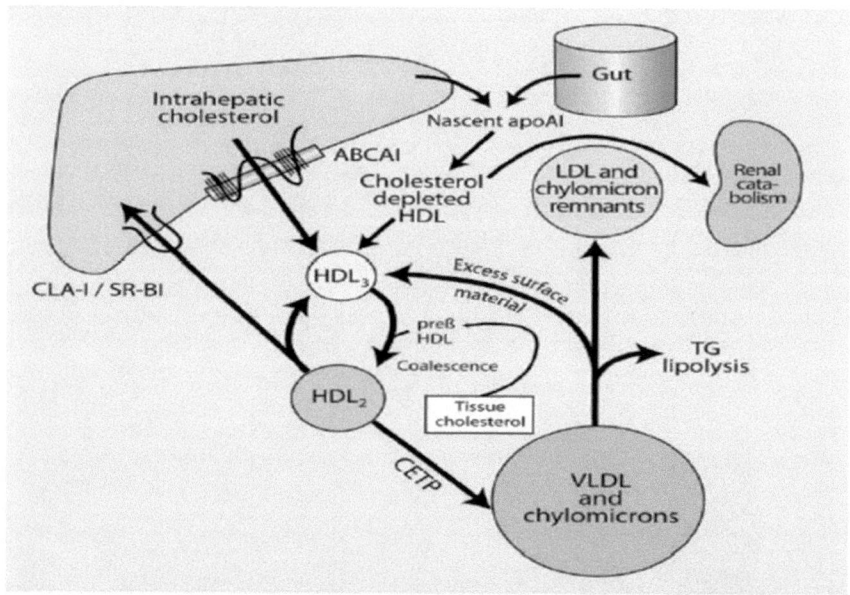

Figure 4: Major influences on circulating HDL levels (Brewer, 2004).

The concentration of ApoA1 and of HDL subfractions observed in plasma is, therefore, a reflection of dynamic processes affecting the structure and function of this lipoprotein class. A major influence on HDL is the metabolic state of triglyceride-rich lipoproteins. Individuals with efficient lipolytic mechanisms clear VLDL and chylomicrons rapidly. Redundant surface phospholipids shed from these delipidated particles, and ApoA1 released from chylomicrons, is transferred to HDL, increasing the potential for particle formation. Likewise, the limited time for exchange of core lipid in people with healthy metabolism leads to a maintenance of high apo AI and cholesterol levels in large HDL particles (Brinton *et al.*, 1994). The converse is true in those with reduced lipolysis rate with the net result that small, dense HDL are formed from which ApoA1 is likely to desorp and be catabolize rapidly (Rye *et al.*, 1999; Lewis and Rader, 2005; Brinton *et al.*, 1994). Metabolic studies have shown a strong inverse relationship between HDL size and Apo AI clearance rates, and a positive association between ApoA1 clearance and plasma triglyceride (Brinton *et al.*, 1994).

Expression of the apoA-I gene is regulated primarily at the transcriptional level. The apo A-I gene promoter contains a TATA-like motif close to the transcriptional start site, while further 5′, several *cis* elements regulate expression of the gene in either a positive or negative manner in response to changes in the hormonal or metabolic status. Expression of the apo A-I gene is subject to regulation by several hormone and metabolic signaling pathways, many of which are altered in diabetes (Arshag *et al.*, 2004). 5′ from the transcriptional start site, an insulin response core element (IRCE) is located between nucleotides -404 and -411 (Murao *et al.*, 1998). This element binds to the ubiquitous transcription factor Sp1 and is responsible for the induction of the apo A-I gene by insulin.

Effect of glucose and insulin on ApoA1 gene expression

Insulin fount to act on the ApoA1 promoter through at least two signaling pathways: Ras-raf and phosphatidylinositol 3-kinase (PI3-K), leading to activation of the mitogen-activated protein kinase (MAPK) and PKC kinases, respectively (Zheng *et al.*, 2000). Despite these differences, all these pathways ultimately target the transcriptional factor Sp1 (Zheng *et al.*, 2000; Samson and Wong, 2002). Cotransfection of Sp1 expression vector with an ApoA1 IRCE reporter construct augments the actions of insulin, while reducing Sp1 levels with an antisense RNA impairs the insulin response (Lam *et al.*, 2003). In addition, experiments with okadaic acid (a cellular phosphatase inhibitor) or other phosphatase inhibitors suggest that phosphorylation of Sp1 plays a critical role in ApoA1 expression by regulating the ability of Sp1 to bind the IRCE. The various molecular signals for Sp1-mediated ApoA1 transcription are summarized in Figure 5 (Samson and Wong, 2002). Indeed, numerous domains at Sp1 are targets for phosphorylation by multiple protein serine/threonine kinases.

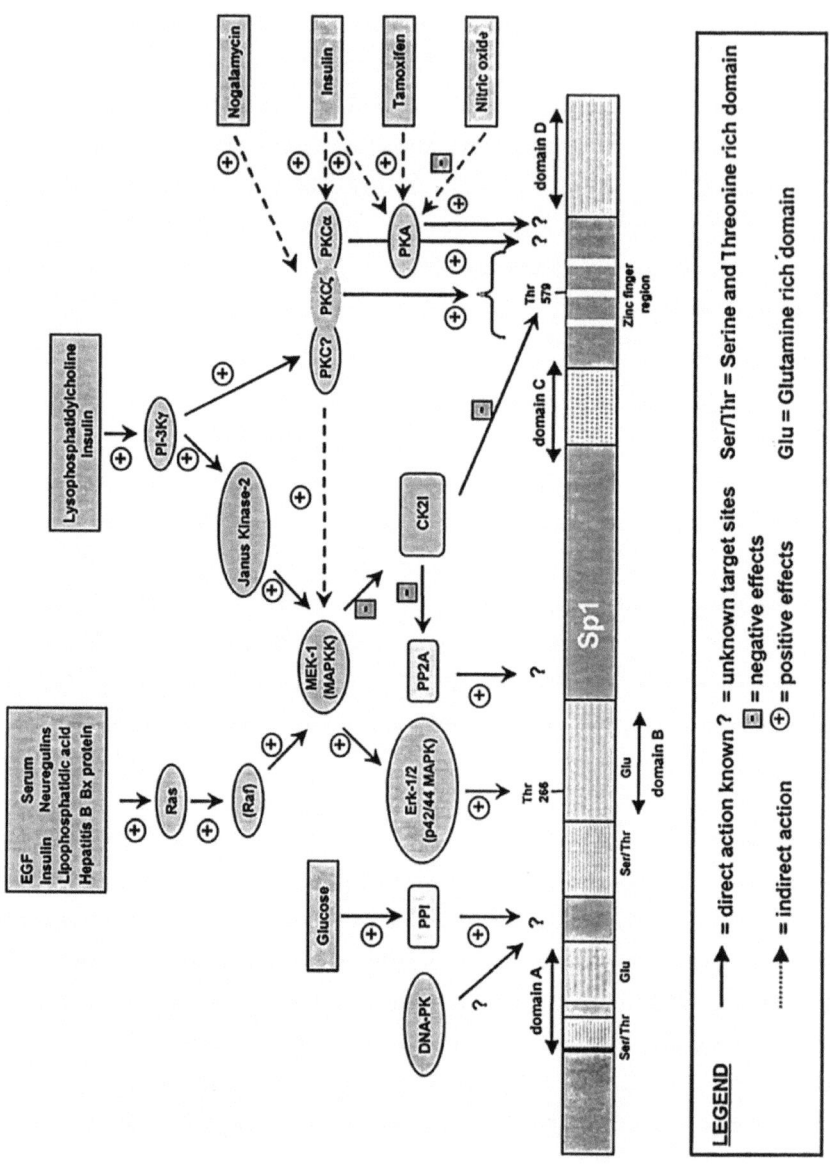

Figure 5. The multiplicity of signaling pathways of Sp1-mediated modulation of gene expression (Arshag *et al.*, 2004).

Effect of insulin resistance on ApoA1 expression

One of the hallmarks of insulin resistance is reduced plasma concentration of HDL cholesterol and low plasma levels of its major apoprotein, namely ApoA1 (Lopez-Candales, 2001; Vajo *et al.*, 2002; Duvillard *et al.*, 2000). This change is mostly attributed to increased fractional clearance of HDL without a change in ApoA1 production (Vajo *et al.*, 2002; Duvillard *et al.*, 2000). However, it is possible that reduced apoA-I expression due to reduced responsiveness of the ApoA1 gene to insulin may contribute to the reduced plasma concentrations of HDL (Arshag *et al.*, 2004). Several regulatory elements mediating numerous transcriptional responses (hormonal, metabolic, and tissue-specific), as well as the factors that mediate both positive and negative effects on ApoA1 gene expression, are shown in Figure 6 (Arshag *et al.*, 2004). In some cases (estradiol, glucocorticoids, and pH), the promoter region modulating the effect has been identified but the factors mediating the process have not been reported. A cytokine response element mediating the suppressive effects of TNF-α and IL-1 is located within site A. TR, thyroid hormone receptor; IRCE/ChRE, insulin response core element/carbohydrate response element; pHRE, pH response element.

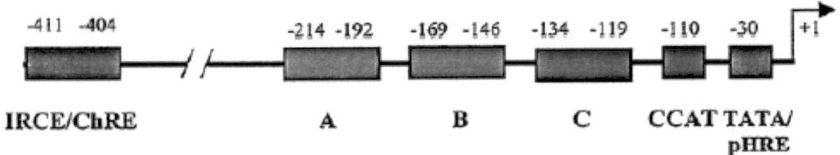

IRCE/ChRE – Sp1
Site A – TR, HNF-4, RARα,β, RXRα, C/EBP,
      ARP-1, PPARα, Rev-erbα
Site B – Glucocorticoids, Estradiol, HNF3β
Site C – HNF-4, ARP-1
TATA – Basal transcriptional apparatus, TR, pH

Figure 6. Organization of regulatory elements within the ApoA1 gene promoter (Arshag *et al.*, 2004).

The reduced expression of ApoA1 in obese T2DM subjects, despite the increased levels of plasma insulin, cannot be simply attributed to insulin resistance. Thus, insulin resistance and hyperinsulinemia induced with a high-fructose diet in rats is associated with increased ApoA1 levels (Mooradian *et al.*, 1997). Similarly, aging in rats is associated with increased expression of ApoA1, although it is accompanied with insulin resistance (Shah *et al.*, 1995). Finally, treatment of hepatocytes with glucosamine, a model of cellular insulin resistance, found to be associated with increased stabilization of ApoA1 mRNA and increased expression of ApoA1 protein (Haas). It appears that the diabetes-related reduction in ApoA1 is not only related to increased plasma clearance of the protein but also is the result of down regulation of ApoA1 expression at a transcriptional level. Although the precise nature for this change is not known, it is likely that increased cytokine production may contribute significantly to the inhibition of ApoA1 gene transcription. The reduced ApoA1 expression in diabetic subjects is due to either reduced responsiveness of the ApoA1 gene to insulin, or secondary to inhibition by the altered metabolic milieu in diabetes, notably increased cytokine production, may contribute to the reduced plasma concentrations of HDL. The myriad of changes that may occur in diabetes, culminating in reduced plasma ApoA1 concentrations, is summarized in Figure 7 (Arshag *et al.*, 2004).

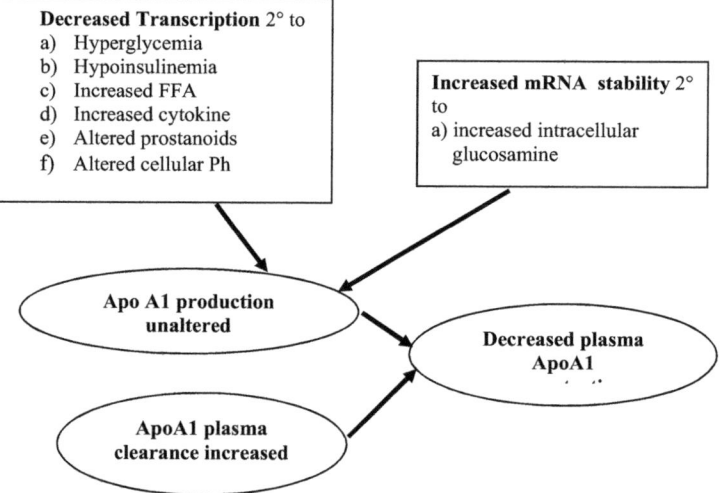

Figure 7. A schematic summary of the myriad of changes that occur in diabetes, culminating in reduced plasma ApoA1 concentrations (Arshag *et al.*, 2004).

Apolipoprotein B

Apolipoprotein B, a major protein component of circulating plasma lipoproteins, exists in 2 forms: ApoB-100 and ApoB-48. The first is synthesized exclusively by the small intestine, the second by the liver. In humans, ApoB-100 is found in lipoproteins originating from the liver (VLDL, IDL and LDL). There is one ApoB-100 molecule per hepatic-derived lipoprotein. ApoB-48 is the form of ApoB present in chylomicrons and chylomicron remnants (Marcovina *et al.*, 2006). Both isoforms are coded by *APOB* and by a single mRNA transcript larger than 16 kb. ApoB-48 is generated when a stop codon (UAA) at residue 2153 is created by RNA editing. There appears to be a *trans*-acting tissue-specific splicing gene that determines which isoform is ultimately produced. Alternatively, there is some evidence that a *cis*-acting element several thousand bp upstream determines which isoform is produced. As a result of the RNA editing, ApoB-48 and ApoB-100 share a common N-terminal sequence, but ApoB-48 lacks Apo-B100's C-terminal LDL receptor binding region.

ApoB-100 is the dominating protein in plasma compared with minute amounts of ApoB-48 even in the postprandial state. Therefore, ApoB is the nomenclature most often used unless specific studies are performed focusing on ApoB-48. ApoB is present in VLDL, IDL, large buoyant LDL and small dense LDL (sd-LDL), with one molecule of ApoB in each of these atherogenic particles (Elovson *et al.*, 1988). Dietary (exogenous) fat is absorbed into chylomicrons (CMs).

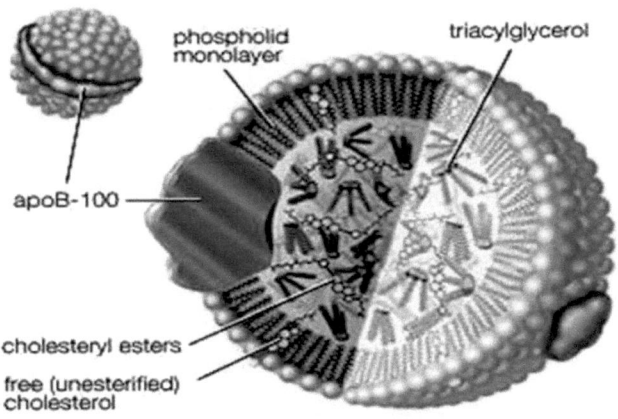

Figure 8: Structure of LDL

In endogenous lipid synthesis, the liver synthesizes triglycerides (TGs) and cholesteryl esters (CEs) and packages them into very-low-density lipoproteins (VLDLs). The enzyme lipoprotein lipase (LPL), bound to the surface of the capillary endothelium (especially in muscle and adipose tissue), hydrolyzes TG in CMs and in VLDLs. Apolipoprotein C-II (ApoC-II), found on CMs, is a required cofactor for LPL. The free fatty acids generated from TG hydrolysis are a source of energy or fat storage, and the resulting CM remnant (CMR) is released and is eventually taken up by the liver. VLDL, which contains the major structural protein ApoB-100, is hydrolyzed by LPL to form intermediate-density lipoprotein (IDL). ApoB stabilizes and allows the transport of cholesterol and TG in plasma VLDL, IDL, large buoyant LDL and sd-LDL. In addition, ApoB serves as the ligand for the ApoB and ApoB, E receptors thereby facilitating uptake of cholesterol in peripheral tissues and the liver (Walldius and Jungner, 2004; Marcovina and Packard, 2006; Sniderman *et al.*, 2003; Sniderman *et al.*, 2006). In most conditions, more than 90% of all ApoB in blood is found in LDL. In cases where LDL C is in the normal/low range, high ApoB levels may indicate an increased number of sd-LDL particles, which are the most atherogenic particles as they are easily oxidized and promote an inflammatory response and the growth of plaques (Walldius and Jungner, 2004; Marcovina and Packard, 2006; Sniderman *et al.*, 2003; Sniderman *et al.*, 2006).

Regulation of plasma apo B levels in normal and dyslipidaemic subjects

Various states of dyslipidaemia are the net result of the processes that regulate lipoprotein production, interconversion and clearance. In normal subjects, although VLDL1 is the main lipoprotein secreted by the liver, its rapid progress down the delipidation cascade means that the concentrations of VLDL1, VLDL2 and IDL in normals are kept low. LDL, on the other hand, is cleared relatively slowly from the circulation (residence time of 2.0–4.0 days; residence time is the reciprocal of fractional catabolic rate) and so it is this species that usually predominates. Lifestyle factors such as obesity promote VLDL synthesis which in turn leads to a rise in LDL and total apo B (Chan *et al.*, 2004), whilst the rise in apoB with age is associated apparently with reduction in the activity of LDL receptors (Matthan *et al.*, 2005).

VLDL1 production is also influenced by insulin levels even in apparently healthy subjects (Malmstrom, 1997). In people with insulin resistance there is failure to regulate properly VLDL production, and apoB levels rise in the VLDL, IDL and LDL density classes (Chan *et al.*, 2004; Taskinen 2003). Individuals with significant hypercholesterolaemia are likely to have raised levels of all apoB containing lipoproteins as a result of reduced clearance of particles by receptors. The LDL receptor is a regulated cell membrane protein responsible for the internalization of lipoproteins by cells that require cholesterol (Turley, 2004). In individuals with hypertriglyceridaemia there is a combination of overproduction of VLDL (especially VLDL1) and inefficient lipolysis (Packard and Shepherd, 1997; Chan *et al.*, 2004). Thus, apo levels are elevated in both VLDL1 and VLDL2. Furthermore, a prolonged residence time in the circulation is seen for all apoB containing lipoproteins which increases the opportunities for these particles to be modified by the processes of inter-particle exchange of lipid and protein components, and by lipolysis.

Mechanisms of VLDL-apoB Overproduction in Insulin Resistant States

A major complication of insulin resistant states, such as T2DM and obesity, is a highly atherogenic lipoprotein and an increased risk of cardiovascular disease (Lakka *et al.*, 2002). The most fundamental defect in these patients is resistance to cellular actions of insulin, particularly resistance to insulin-stimulated glucose uptake. Insulin insensitivity appears to cause hyperinsulinemia, enhanced hepatic gluconeogenesis and glucose output and reduced suppression of lipolysis in adipose tissue leading to high free fatty acid flux, and increased VLDL secretion causing hypertriglyceridemia (Reaven, 1992; Lewis and Steiner, 1996; Kissebah, 1991; Grundy *et al.*, 1979). Binding of insulin to the insulin receptor triggers signaling mechanisms that negatively regulate VLDL assembly and secretion principally via the PI-3 kinase pathway. This negative regulation appears to be lost in insulin resistant states leading to stimulation of VLDL production. Upregulation of key phosphatases, including PTP-1B and PTEN, may play an important role in downregulation of PI-3 kinase signaling.

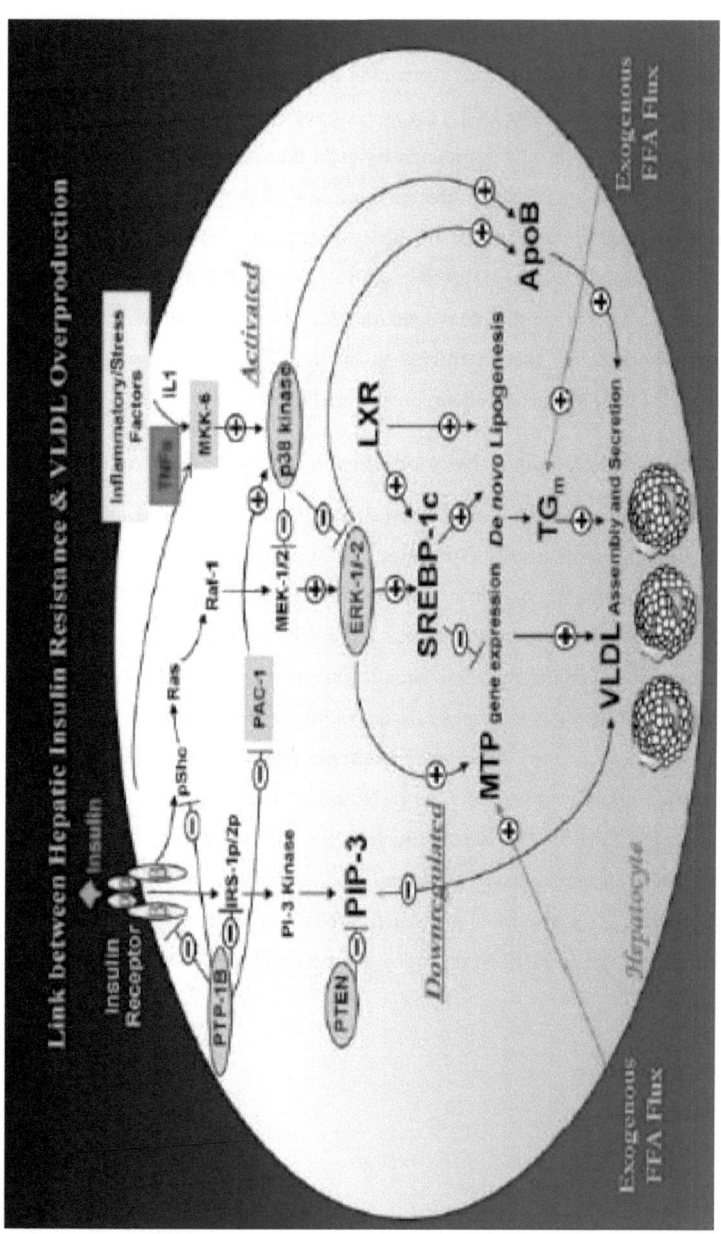

Figure 9: Molecular mechanisms linking insulin resistance and metabolic dyslipidemia (Avramoglu and Adeli, 2004).

Conversely, inflammatory and stress mechanisms result in stimulation of the MAP kinase pathway which in turn can upregulate MTP, SREBP-1c, and ApoB, leading to increased de novo lipogenesis and enhanced VLDL secretion. Increased free fatty acid flux into the liver in the insulin resistant state also plays an important role in MTP activation and enhanced triglyceride synthesis that contribute to VLDL production and thus exacerbate elevated circulating VLDL (Avramoglu and Adeli, 2004).

Insulin and apolipoproteins

Hyperinsulinemia is associated with adverse changes in apolipoprotein levels, particularly an increase in apolipoprotein (apo) B and a decrease in apoAI concentration. (Hunt *et al.*, 1989; Wing *et al.*, 1989). Insulin could alter the activity of lipid transfer protein which is particularly pronounced after meals and is affected by HDL composition (Patsch *et al.*, 1983). Whether insulin promotes hepatic VLDL secretion remains controversial (Reaven 1967; Durrington 1982). Hyperinsulinemia can acutely inhibit VLDL ApoB secretion in normal subjects (but not in obese insulin-resistant subjects) (Lewis *et al.*, 1993). Hyperglycemia arising from hypo-or hyperinsulinemic states such as diabetes decreases the levels of apo A-1 (Barrett-Connor *et al.*, 1987). Experiments showed that in the hyperinsulinemic and hyperglycemic animals, an enhancement of the VLDL assembly machinery was responsible for the increased levels of plasma lipoproteins observed (Zoltowska *et al.*, 2004 and 2001). Peripheral hyperinsulinemia, due to either insulin-treated diabetes mellitus or insulinoma, will usually lead to reductions in VLDL and LDL with increased HDL lipid (Taskinen *et al.*, 1988 Winocour *et al.*, 1985; Golay *et al.*, 1987). Hepatic insulin insensitivity alters both lipoprotein synthetic and lipoprotein catabolic rates in the liver (Winocour *et al.*, 1992). Stewart et al (1998) have shown that first-degree relatives of diabetic patients had increased apoB and decreased apoA-I values and that they were more obese and will be more insulin-resistant, but normoglycaemic, than age- and sex-matched controls.

REFERENCES

Acton S, Rigotti A, Landschulz KT, Xu S, Hobbs HH, Krieger M. Identification of scavenger receptor SR-BI as a high-density lipoprotein receptor. *Science* 1996; **271**:518–520.

Al-Bahrani AI, Bakhiet CS, Bayoumi RA, Al-Yakyaee SA. A potential role of apolipoprotein B in the risk stratification of diabetic patients with dyslipidaemia. *Diabetes Res Clin Pract* 2005; **69**: 44–51.

Albers JJ, Wahl PW, Cabana VG, Hazzard WR, Hoover JJ: Quantitation of apolipoprotein A-I of human high density Iipoprotein. *Metabolism* 1976; **25**:633-644.

American Diabetes Association (ADA). Report of the expert committee on the diagnosis and classification of diabetes mellitus. *Diabetes Care* 1997; **20**: 1183-1197.

American Diabetic Association (ADA). Diagnosis and classification of diabetic mellitus. *Diabetes care* 2005; **28**: 37-42.

Anderson JW, Kendall CW, Jenkins DJ. Importance of weight management in type 2 diabetes review with meta-analysis of clinical studies. *J Am Coll Nutr* 2003; **22**: 331–339.

Arad Y., Ramakrishnan R., Ginsberg H. N. Lovastatin therapy reduces low density lipoprotein apoB levels in subjects with combined hyperlipidemia by reducing the production of apoB-containing lipoproteins: implications for the pathophysiology of apoB production. *J. Lipid Res.* 1990; **31**,567–582

Arshag D. Mooradian, Michael J H, Norman C W W. Transcriptional Control of Apolipoprotein A-I Gene Expression in Diabetes. *Diabetes* 2004; **53**:513-520.

Balkau B and Eschwege E. The diagnosis and classification of diabetes and impaired glucose regulation. In: *Text book of diabetes*, third edition , John C, Pickup & Gareth Williams, Eds, Blackwell science, 2003,2.1-2.13.

Barter P, Kastelein J, Nunn A, Hobbs R. Future Forum Editorial Board. High density lipoproteins (HDL) and atherosclerosis; the unanswered questions. *Atherosclerosis* 2003; **168**: 195–2.

Barter P. J., Ballantyne C. M., Carmena R., CabezasM. C, Chapman M. J, Couture P.et al. Report of the thirty person/ten country panel. ApoB versus cholesterol to estimate cardiovascular risk and to guide therapy. *J Intern Med* 2006; **259**: 247–58.

Barter PJ, Rye K-A. The rationale for using apoA-I as a clinical marker of cardiovascular risk. *J Intern Med* 2006;**259**: 447–54.

Bergenstal RM, Kendall DM, Franz MJ, et al. Endocrinology. W.B. Saunders, 2001; P. 810-20.

Bergman RN, Finegood DT, Kahn SE. The evolution of ß-cell dysfunction and insulin resistance in type 2 diabetes. *European J Clin Invest* 2002; **32:35**-45.

Berneis KK, Krauss RM. Metabolic origins and clinical significance of LDL heterogeneity. *J Lipid Res* 2002; **43**: 1363–79.

Boronat M, et al., *Diabetes Medicine* 2002;**19**: 558-565(8).

Bourgeois CS, Wiggins D, Hems R, Gibbons GF. VLDL output by hepatocytes from obese Zucker rats is resistant to the inhibitory effect of insulin. *Am J Physiol* 1995; **269**:E208-E215.

Breslow JL. Familial disorders of high-density lipoprotein metabolism. In: Scriver CR, Beaudet AL, Sly WS, Valle D, eds. *The Metabolic and Molecular Bases of Inherited Disease.* 7th ed. New York: McGraw-Hill; 1995:2031–2052.

Brewer HB. High-density lipoproteins: a new potential therapeutic target for the prevention of cardiovascular diseases. *Arterioscler Thromb Vasc Biol* 2004; **24**: 387–91.

Brinton EA, Eisenberg S, Breslow JL. Human HDL C levels are determined by apo AI fractional catabolic rate, which correlates inversely with estimates of HDL particle size. Effects of gender, hepatic and lipoprotein lipases, triglyceride and insulin levels and body fat distribution. *Arterioscler Thromb Vasc Biol* 1994; **14**: 707–20.

Brunzell JD. Familial lipoprotein lipase deficiency and other causes of the chylomicronemia syndrome. In: Scriver CR, Beaudet AL, Sly WS, Valle D, eds. *The Metabolic and Molecular Bases of Inherited Disease.* 7th ed. New York: McGraw-Hill; 1995:1913–1932.

Chan DC, Bennet PHR, Watts GF. Dyslipidemia in visceral obesity: mechanisms, implications and therapy. *Am J Cardiovasc Drugs* 2004; **4**: 227–46.

Christison JK, Rye KA, Stocker R. Exchange of oxidized cholesteryl linoleate between LDL and HDL mediated by cholesteryl ester transfer protein. *J Lipid Res* 1995; **36:2017**-2026.

Corpeleijn E, Mensink M, Feskens EJM, de Bruin TWA, Saris WHM, Blaak EE. Prevalence of glucose intolerance in a Dutch population at risk: impact of sex, age and Body mass index, [Online], Available from : http://212.144.4.93/easd/customfiles /easd/38th/abstract/PS5.htm[May7, 2006]

Crepaldi G, Tienzo A, Baggio G (eds): Diabetes, Obesity and Hyperlipidaemia. *Excerpta Medica*, International Congress Series 1985; **681**:269-270.

Dashti N, Williams DL, Alaupovic P: Effects of oleate and insulin on the production and cellular mRNA concentrations of apolipoproteins in HepG2 cells. *J Lipid Res* 1989; **30**:1365-1373.

Dashti N, Wolfbauer G: Secretion of lipids, apolipoproteins, and lipoproteins by human hepatoma cell line, HepG2: Effects of oleic acid and insulin. *Lipid Res* 1987; **8**:423-426

Davies MJ, Raymond NT, Day JL, Hales CN, Burden AC. Impaired glucose tolerance and fasting hyperglycemia have different characteristics. *Diabet Med* 2000; **17**:433-440.

DeFronzo RA, Ferrannini E, Simonson DC. J Fasting hyperglycemia in non-insulin-dependent diabetes mellitus: contributions of excessive hepatic glucose production and impaired tissue glucose uptake. *Metabolism* 1989;**38**: 387-95.

DeFronzo RA. Lilly Lecture. The triumvirate: beta cell, muscle, liver. A collusion responsible for NIDDM. *Diabetes* 1988; **37**: 667-687.

Dowse GK, Zimmet PZ, Collins VR. Insulin levels and the natural history of glucose intolerance in Nauruans. *Diabetes* 1996; **45**:1367-1372.

Duvillard L, Pont F, Florentin E, Gambert P, Verges B: Inefficiency of insulin therapy to correct apolipoprotein A-I metabolic abnormalities in non-insulin-dependent diabetes mellitus. *Atherosclerosis* 2000;**152**:229–237.

Eckel RH: Lipoprotein lipase: A multifunctional enzyme relevant to common metabolic diseases. *N Engl J Med* 1989; **320**:1060-1068.

Eisenberg S. High-density lipoprotein metabolism. *J Lipid Res* 1984;**25**:1017–1058.

Elovson J, Chatterton JE, Bell GT, Schumaker VN, Reuben MA, Puppione DL, Reeve JR Jr, Young NL..et al Plasma very low density lipoproteins contain a single molecule of apolipoprotein B. *J Lipid Res* 1988; **29**: 1461–73.

Eriksson J, Franssila-Kallunki A, Ekstrand A, Saloranta C, Widen E, Schalin C, Groop L. Early metabolic defects in persons at increased risk for non-insulin-dependent diabetes mellitus. *New Engl J Med* 1989; **321**:337-343.

Eriksson M, Carlson LA, Miettinen TA, Angelin B. Stimulation of fecal steroid excretion after infusion of recombinant proapolipoprotein AI. Potential reverse cholesterol transport in humans. *Circulation* 1999; **100**: 594–8.

Erkelens DW. Apolipoproteins in lipid transport, an iznpressionist view. *Postgrad Med J* 1989; **65**:275-81.

Festa A, D'Agostino R J, Hanley AJG, Karter AJ, Saad MF and Haffner SM. Difference in insulin resistance in nondiabetic subjects with isolated impaired glucose tolerance and impaired fasting glucose. *Diabetes* 2004; **53**: 1549-1555.

Fielding CJ, Fielding PE. Molecular physiology of reverse cholesterol transport. *J Lipid Res* 1995;**36**:211–228.

Fossati P; Prencipe L. Serum triglyceride determined colourimatrically with an enzyme that produce hydrogen peroxide. *Clin Chem*1982; **28**: 2077.

Friedewald WT, Levy RI and Fredrickson DS. Estimation of the concentration of lowdenspy lipoprotein cholesterol in plasma, with the use of preparative centrifuge. *Clin Chem* 1972;**18**:499-502.

Gaffney D, Forster L, Caslake MJ, Bedford D, Stewart JP, Stewart G et al. Comparison of apolipoprotein B metabolism in familial defective apolipoprotein B and heterozygous familial hypercholesterolemia. *Atherosclerosis* 2002; **162**: 33–43.

Garner B, Waldeck AR, Witting PK, Rye KA, Stocker R. Oxidation of high density lipoproteins. II. Evidence for direct reduction of lipid hydroperoxides by methionine residues of apolipoproteins AI and AII. *J Biol Chem* 1998;**273**:6088-6095.

Ginsberg HN. Insulin resistance and cardiovascular disease. *J. Clin. Invest* 2000; **106**: 453–458

Golay A, Zech L, Shi M-Z, Jeng C-Y, Chiou Y-AM, Reaven GM,Chen Y-DI: Role of insulin in regulation of high density Iipoprotein metabolism. *J Lipid Res* 1987; **28**:10-18.

Gordon T, Castelli WP, Hjertland M, Kannel WB, Dawber TR:Diabetes, blood lipids and the role of obesity in coronary heart disease risk for women: The Framingham study. *Ann Intern Med* 1977; **83**:393-397.

Grundy SM, Mok HY, Zech L, Steinberg D, Berman M. Transport of very low density lipoprotein triglycerides in varying degrees of obesity and hypertriglyceridemia. *J Clin Invest* 1979; **63**:1274–1283.

Haas MJ, Wong NCW, Mooradian AD: Effect of glucosamine on apolipoprotein

Haffner SM, Miettinen H, Gaskill SP, Stern MP. Decreased insulin secretion and increased insulin resistance are independently related to the 7-year risk of NIDDM in Mexican-Americans. *Diabetes* 1995; **44**:1386-1391.

Haffner SM, Miettinen H, Stern MP. Insulin secretion and resistance in nondiabetic Mexican Americans and non-Hispanic whites with a parental history of diabetes. *J Clin Endocrinol Metab* 1996; **81**:1846-1851.

Hanfeld M, Koehler C, Fuecker k, Henkel K, Schaper F, Temelkova- Kurktschiev T. Insulin secretion and insulin sensitivity pattern is different in isolated impaired glucose tolersnce and impaired fasting glucose. *Diabetes Care* 2003;26: 868-874.

Hansen BC, Bodkin NH. Heterogeneity of insulin responses: phases leading to type 2 (noninsulin-dependent) diabetes mellitus in the rhesus monkey. *Diabetologia* 1986; **29**:713-719.

Harris MI. Diabetes Mellitus: *A Fundamental and Clinical Text*. Lippincott Williams & Wilkins, Philadelphia, USA, 2000; pp: 326-34.

Havel RJ. Remnant lipoproteins as therapeutic targets. *Curr Opin Lipidol* 2000; **15**: 615–20.

Hussain MM, Zannis VI. Intracellular modification of human apolipoprotein AII (apoAII) and sites of apoII synthesis: comparison of apoAII with apoCII and apoCII isoproteins. *Biochemistry* 1990; **29**:209–217.

International Diabetes Federation (IDF). *Diabetes Atlas*. 2nd Edition. Gan D ed. 2003.Brussels, Belgium.

Jallut D, Golay A, Munger R, Frascarolo P, Schutz Y, Jequier E, Felber JP. Impaired glucose tolerance and diabetes in obesity: a 6 year follow-up study of glucose metabolism. *Metabolism* 1990;**39**:1068-1075.

Jensen CC, Cnop M, Hull RL, Fujimoto WY, Kahn SE, the American Diabetes Association GENNID Study Group. ß-cell function is a major contributor to oral glucose tolerance in high-risk relatives of our ethnic groups in the U.S. *Diabetes* 2002; **51**:2170-2178.

Jensen E, Floren C-H, Nilsson A: Insulin stimulates the uptake of chylomicron remnants in cultured rat hepatocytes. *EurJ Clin Invest* 1985; **28**:412-419.

Kabir F. Association of serum visfatin and plasma retinol binding protein 4 with insulin secretion and sensitivity among prediabetic subjects. MPhil(Medical Biochemistry) thesis 2008. BIRDEM academy, University of Dhaka, Bangladesh.

Kahn SE. Clinical Review 135. The importance of ß-cell failure in the development and progression of type 2 diabetes. *J Clin Endocrinol Metab* 2001;**86**:4047-4058.

Kane, J. P., *Method. Enzymol.* 1986;**129**:123-129.

Kasim S, Tseng K, Jen K-L, Khilnani S: Significance of hepatic triglyceride lipase activity in the regulation of serum high density lipoproteins in type II diabetes mellitus. *J CUn Endocrinol Metab* 1987; **65**:183-187.

Kim BJ, Hwang ST, Sung KC, Kim BS, Kang JH, Lee MH et al. Comparison of the relationships between serum apolipoprotein B and serum lipid distributions. *Clin Chem* 2005; **51**: 2257–63.

Kim HK, Chang SA, Choi EK, Kim YJ, Kim HS, Sohn DW, et al. Association between plasma lipids, and apolipoproteins and coronary artery disease: a cross-sectional study in a low-risk Korean population. *Int J Cardiol* 2005; **101**: 435-40.

Kissebah AH. Insulin resistance in visceral obesity. *Int J Obes* 1991; **15** :109–115.

Knowler WC, Barrett-Connor E, Fowler SE, et al.: Diabetes Prevention Program Research Group. Reduction in the incidence of type 2 diabetes with lifestyle intervention or metformin. *N Engl J Med* 2002, **346**:393-403.

Lakka HM, Laaksonen DE, Lakka TA, Niskanen LK, Kumpusalo E, Tuomilehto J, Salonen JT. The metabolic syndrome and total and cardiovascular disease mortality in middle-aged men. *JAMA* 2002; **288**:2709–2716.

Lam JK, Matsubara S, Mihara K, Zheng X, Mooradian AD, Wong NCW. Insulin induction of apolipoprotein A: role of SP1. *Biochemistry* 2003; **42**:2680–2690.

Levy et al. Correct Homeostasis Model Assessment (HOMA) Evaluation uses the computer program. *Diabetes Care* 1998; 21: 2191–2.

Lewis GF, Rader DJ. New insights into the regulation of HDL metabolism and reverse cholesterol transport. *Circ Res* 2005; **96**: 122–32

Lewis GF, Steiner G. Acute effects of insulin in the control of VLDL production in humans. Implications for the insulin-resistant state. *Diabetes Care* 1996; **19**:390–393.

Lewis GF, Uffelman KD, Szeto LW, Steiner G. Effects of acute hyperinsulinemia on VLDL triglyceride and VLDL apoB production in normal weight and obese individuals. *Diabetes* 1993;**42**:833-842.

Lewis GF. Fatty acid regulation of very low density lipoprotein (VLDL) production. *Curr Opin Lipidol* 1999;**10**:475-477.

Li CL, Tsai ST and Chou P. Relative role of insulin resistance and B-cell dysfunction in the progression to type 2 diabetes- The Kinmen Study. *Diab Res Clin Pract* 2003; **59**: 225-232.

Lillioja S, Mott DM, Howard BV,Bennett PH, Yki-Jarvinen H, Freymond D, Nyomba BL, Zurlo F, Swinburn B, Bogardus C. Impaired glucose tolerance as a disorder of insulin action. Longitudinal and cross-sectional studies in Pima Indians. *New Engl J Med* 1988;**318**: 1217-25.

Lind L, Vessby B, Sundstro¨m J. The apolipoprotein B/AI ratio and the metabolic syndrome independently predict risk for myocardial infarction in middle-aged men. *Arterioscler Thromb Vasc Biol* 2006; **26**: 406–10.

Liu J, Sempos C, Donahue RP, Dorn J, Trevisan M, Grundy SM. Joint distribution of non-HDL and LDL cholesterol and coronary heart disease risk prediction among individuals with and without diabetes. *Diabetes Care* 2005; **28**: 1916–21.

Lopez-Candales. A Metabolic syndrome X: a comprehensive review of the pathophysiology and recommended therapy. *J Med* 2001; **32**:283–300.

Low-Beer TS, Wicks ACB, Heaton KW, Durrington PN, Yeates J: Fluctuations of serum and bile lipid concentrations during the normal menstrual cycle. *Br Med J* 1977; I:1568-1570.

Mahtab H, Ibrahim M, Banik NG, Gulshan- E-Jahan, Ali SMK. Diabetes detection survey in a rural and semiurban community in Bangladesh. *Tohoku J Exp Med* 1983; **141**: 211–217.

Malmstrom R, Packard CJ, Caslake M, et al. Defective regulation of triglyceride metabolism by insulin in the liver in NIDDM. *Diabetologia* 1997; **40**:454-462.

Malmstrom R; Packard C J.; Watson T.; Rannikko S; Caslake M; Bedford D; et al. Metabolic basis of hypotrigyceridemic effects of insulin in normal men. Arterioscler *Thromb Vasc Biol* 1997; **17**: 1456–64

Marcovina S, Packard CJ. Measurement and meaning of apolipoprotein AI and apolipoprotein B plasma levels. *J Intern Med* 2006; **259**: 437–46.

Matthan NR, Jalbert SM, Lamon-Fava S, Dolnikowski GG, Welty FK, Barrett HR, Schaefer EJ,et al. TRL, IDL and LDL apolipoprotein B and HDL apolipoprotein AI kinetics as a function of age and menopausal status. *Arterioscler Thromb Vasc Biol* 2005; **25**: 1691–6.

Mooradian AD, Wong NCW, Shah GN: Apolipoprotein A1 expression in young and aged rats is modulated by dietary carbohydrates. *Metabolism* 46:1132–1136, 1997.

Murao K, Wada Y, Nakamura T, Taylor AH, Mooradian AD, Wong NCW. Effects of glucose and insulin on rat apolipoprotein A-I gene expression. *J Biol Chem* 1998; **273**:18959–18965.

Packard CJ, Demant T, Stewart JP, Bedford D,. Caslake M J, Schwertfeger G, et al. Apolipoprotein B metabolism and the distribution of VLDL and LDL subfractions. *J Lipid Res* 2000; **41**: 205–18.

Packard CJ, Shepherd J. Lipoprotein heterogeneigty and apolipoprotein B metabolism. *Arterioscler Thromb Vasc Biol* 1997; **17**: 3542–556.

Packard CJ, Shepherd J. Lipoprotein heterogeneigty and apolipoprotein B metabolism. *Arterioscler Thromb Vasc Biol* 1997; **17**: 3542–556.

Peter H. Winocour, Samuel Kaluvya, Kaushik Ramaiya, Linda Brown, Jill P. Millar, Martyn arrer, et al Relation Between Insulinemia, Body Mass Index, and Lipoprotein Composition in Healthy, Nondiabetic Men and Women Arterioscler. *Thromb. Vasc. Biol* 1992;**12**;393-402.

Rader DJ, Hoeg JM, Brewer HB Jr. Quantitation of plasma apolipoproteins in the primary and secondary prevention of coronary artery disease. *Ann Intern Med* 1994;**120**: 1012–25.

Rader DJ. Lipid disorders. In: Topol EJ, ed. *Textbook of Cardiovascular Medicine*. Philadelphia: Lippincott-Raven; 1998:59–90.

Rahman M H, Hafizur R M, Huq F, Nahar Q, Tazib T, Khan A R, Ali L. Insulin secretion and insulin sensitivity in subjects with IGR. *Diabetologia* 2006; **49**: 451.

Rasmussen SS, Glumer S, Sandbaek A, Lauritzen T, Borch- Johnsen K: Progression from Impaired Fasting Glucose and Impaired Glucose Tolerance to diabetes in a high-risk screening programme in general practice: the addition study, Denmark, *Diabetologia* 2007;**50**: 293-297.

Reaven GM, Chen YD, Jeppesen J, Maheux P, Krauss RM. Insulin resistance and hyperinsulinemia in individuals with small, dense low density lipoprotein particles. *J Clin Invest* 1993; **92**:141–146.

Reaven GM, Hollenbeck C, Jeng C-Y, Wu MS, Chen Y-DI: Measurement of plasma glucose, free fatty acid, lactate insulin for 24 h in patients with NIDDM. *Diabetes* 1988; **37**:1020-1024.

Reaven GM. The role of insulin resistance and hyperinsulinemia in coronary heart disease. *Metabolism* 1992; **41**:16–19.

Richmond W. Quantitative determination of cholesterol in serum or plasma by enzymatic method. *Clin Chem* 1973; 19: 1350

Rita Kohen Avramoglu and Khosrow Adeli. *Reviews in Endocrine & Metabolic Disorders* 2004;**5**:293–301.

Rye KA, Clay MA, Barter PJ. Remodelling of high density lipoproteins by plasma factors. *Atherosclerosis* 1999;**145**:227-238.

Saad MF, Knowler WC, Pettitt DJ, Nelson RG, Mott DM, Bennett PH. Sequential changes in serum insulin concentration during development of non-insulin-dependent diabetes. *Lancet* 1989; i:1356-1359.

Saad MF, Knowler WC, Pettitt DJ, Nelson RG, Mott DM, Bennett PH. The natural history of impaired glucose tolerance in the Pima Indians. *New Engl J Med* 1988; **319**:1500-1505.

Samson SL, Wong NC. Role of Sp1 in insulin regulation of gene expression. *J Mol Endocrinol* 2002; **29**:265–279.

Sayeed MA, Hussain MZ, Banu A, Ali L, Rumi MAK, Azad Khan AK: Effect of socioeconomic risk factor on difference between rural and urban in the prevalence of diabetes in Bangladesh. *Diabetes Care* 1997;**20**:551–555.

Sayeed MA, Hussain MZ, Banu A, Rumin MAK, Azad Khan AK: Prevalence of diabetes in a suburban population of Bangladesh. *Diabetes Res Clin Pract* 1997; **34:149**–155.

Sayeed MA, Khan AR, Banu A, Hussain MZ: Prevalence of diabetes and hypertension in a rural population of Bangladesh. *Diabetes Care* 1995;**18**:555–558.

Schianca GPC, Rossi A, Sainaghi pp, Maduli E and Bartoli E. The significance of IFG versus IGT: Importance of Insulin Secretion and resistance. *Diabetes care* 2003; **26**: 1333-1337.

Schlitt A, Blankenberg S, Bickel C, Meyer J, Hafner G, Jiang XC, et al. Prognostic value of lipoproteins and their relation to inflammatory markers among patients with coronary artery disease. *Int J Cardiol* 2005; **102**: 477–85.

Segrest, J. P.,Garber, D. W., Brouillette, C. G., Harvey, S. C., Anantharamaiah, G. M. AdV. *Protein Chem* 1994; **45**:303-369.

Shah NG, Wong NCW, Mooradian AD: Age-related changes in apolipoprotein A-I expression. *Biochim Biophys Acta* 1995;**1259**:277–282.

Shah PK, Kaul S, Nilsson J, Cercek B. Exploiting the vascular protective effects of high-density lipoprotein and its apolipoproteins. An idea whose time for testing is coming: Part I. *Circulation* 2001; **104**: 2376–83.

Sharp DS, Burchfield CM, Rodriguez BL, Sharrett AR, Sorlie PD, Marcovina SM. Apolipoprotein A-I predicts coronary heart disease only at low concentrations of high-density lipoprotein cholesterol: an epidemiological study of Japanese-Americans. *Int J Clin Lab Res* 2000; **30**: 39–48.

Shaw JE, Zimmet PZ, de Courten M, Dowse GK, Chitson P, Gareeboo H, *et al.* Impaired fasting glucose or impaired glucose tolerance. What best predicts future diabetes in Mauritius. *Diabetes Care* 1999; **22**: 399–402.

Shepherd J, Packard CJ, Patsch JR, Gotto AM, Taunton OD: Metabolism of apolipoproteins A-I and A-II and its influence on high density lipoprotein distribution in males and females. *Eur J Clin Invest* 1978; **8**:115-120.

Shefin SM. Insulin Secretion and Insulin Sensitivity in First Degree Relatives of Subjects with Impaired Glucose Regulation. MD (Endocrinology and Metabolism) Thesis 2007; University of Dhaka.

Sicree R, Shaw J, Zimmet P. The global burden of diabetes. In *"Diabetes Atlas"*. 2nd ed. Gan D, Ed. Brussels, International Diabetes Federation 2003; pp. 15–71.

Sierra-Johnson J, Romero-Corral A, Somers VK, Lopez-Jimenez F, Walldius G, Hamsten A. *et al.* ApoB/apoA-I ratio: an independent predictor of insulin resistance in us non-diabetic subjects. European Heart Journal 2007; **28**: 2637-2643.

Skinner JS, Farrer M, Albers CJ, Neil HA, Adams PC. High apolipoprotein AI concentrations are associated with lower mortality and myocardial infarction five years after coronary artery bypass graft surgery. *Heart* 1999; **81**: 488–94.

Smith J, Amri MA, Sniderman AD. What do we (not) know about apoB, type 2 diabetes and obesity. *Diabetes Res Clin Pract* 2005; **69**: 99–101.

Snehalatha C, Ramachandran A, Sivasankari S, Satyavani K, Viswanathan V, Misra J, et al. Is increased apolipoprotein B-A major factor enhancing the risk coronary artery disease in type 2 diabetes? *J Assoc Physicians India* (JAPI) 2002; **50**: 1036–8.

Sniderman AD, Furberg CD, Keech A, Roeters van Lennep JE, Frohlich J, Jungner I, Walldius G.et al.,. Apolipoproteins versus lipids as indices of coronary risk and as targets for statin therapy treatment. *Lancet* 2003; **361**: 777–80.

Sniderman AD, Scantlebury T, Cianflone K. Hypertriglyceridemic hyperapoB: the unappreciated atherogenic dyslipoproteinemia in type 2 diabetes mellitus. *Ann Intern Med* 2001; **135**: 447–59.

Solymoss BC, Bourassa MG, Campeau L et al. Effect of increasing metabolic syndrome score on atherosclerotic risk profile and coronary artery disease angiographic severity. *Am J Cardiol* 2004; **93**: 159–64.

Songer TJ, Zimmet P. *Pharmacoeconomics* 1995; **1**:1-11.

Sparks JD, Sparks CE. Insulin regulation of triacylglycerol-rich lipoprotein synthesis and secretion. *Biochim Biophys Acta* 1994; **1215**:9-32.

Stalder M, Pometta D, Suenram A: Relationship between plasma insulin levels and high density lipoprotein cholesterol levels in healthy men. *Diabetologia* 1981; **21**:544-548.

Stern MP and Burke JP. Impaired glucose tolerance and impaired fasting glucose –Risk factors or Diagnostic categories. In: Diabetes Mellitus: *A fundamental and clinical text*, 2nd edition, Derek Leroith, Simeon I. Taylor and Jerrold M Olefsky, Eds, Lippincott Williams & Wilkins, 2000, 558-595.

Stewart MW, Humphriss DB, Mitcheson J, Webster J, Walker M, Laker MF. Lipoprotein composition and serum apolipoproteins in normoglycaemic first-degree relatives of noninsulin dependent diabetic patients. *Atherosclerosis* 1998; **139**: 115–21.

Sung KC, Hwang ST. Association between insulin resistance and apolipoprotein B in normoglycemic Koreans. *Atherosclerosis* 2005; **189**: 161–9.

Taghibiglou C, Rashid-Kolvear F, Van Iderstine SC, et al. Hepatic very low density lipoprotein-ApoB overproduction is associated with attenuated hepatic insulin signaling and overexpression of protein-tyrosine phosphatase 1B in a fructose-fed hamster model of insulin resistance. *J Biol Chem* 2002; **277**:793-803.

Taskinen M-R, Kuusi T, Helve E, Nikkila EA, Yki-Jarvinen H: Insulin therapy induces antiatherogenic changes of serum lipoproteins in non-insulin dependent diabetes. *Atherosclerosis* 1988; **8**: 168-177.

Taskinen M-R, Nikkila EA: Lipoprotein lipase activity of adipose tissue and skeletal muscle in insulin-deficient human diabetes: Relation to high density and very low density lipoprotein and response to treatment. *Diabetologia* 1979; **17**:351-356.

Taskinen MR. Diabetic dyslipidaemia from basic research to clinical practice. *Diabetologia* 2003; **46**: 733–49.

Taskinen MR. Insulin resistance and lipoprotein metabolism. *Curr Opin Lipidol* 1995; **6**:153–160.

Tripathy D, Carlsson M, Almgren P, Osomaa B, Raskinen M-R, Tuomi T, Groop LC. Insulin secretion and insulin sensitivity in relation to glucose tolerance. Lessons from the Botnia Study. *Diabetes* 2000;**49**:975-980.

Trinder P. *Ann Clin Biochem* 1969; **6**: 24.

Tripathy D, Carlsson M, Almgren P, Osomaa B, Raskinen M-R, Tuomi T, Groop LC. Insulin secretion and insulin sensitivity in relation to glucose tolerance. Lessons from the Botnia Study. *Diabetes* 49:975-980, 2000.

Tsunoda T, Tuzcu EM, Schoenhagen P, Cooper CJ, Yasin M et al. Effect of recombinant ApoA-I Milano on coronary atherosclerosis in patients with acute coronary syndromes. A randomized controlled trial. *Am Med Assoc* 2003;**290**: 2292–300.

Tuomilehto J, Lindstrom J, Eriksson JG, Valle TT, Hamalainen H, Ilanne-Parikka P, Keinanen-Kiukaanniemi S, Laakso M, Louheranta A, Rastas M, et al.: Prevention of type 2 diabetes mellitus by changes in lifestyle among subjects with impaired glucose tolerance. *N Engl J Med* 2001, **344**:1343-1350.

Turley SD. Cholesterol metabolism and therapeutic targets: rationale for multiple metabolic pathways. *Clin Cardiol* 2004; **27**: III16–21.

Unwin N, Shaw J, Zimmet P, Alberti KGMM. Impaired glucose tolerance and impaired fasting glycemia: the current status on definition and intervention. *Diabetic Medicine* 2002; **19**: 708-723.

Vaag A, Henriksen JE, Beck-Nielsen. Decreased insulin activation of glycogen synthase in skeletal muscles in young non-obese Caucasian first-degree relatives of patients with non-insulin-dependent diabetes mellitus. *J Clin Invest* 1992; **89**:782-788.

Vajo Z, Terry JG, Brinton EA: Increased intra-abdominal fat may lower HDL levels by increasing the fractional catabolic rate of Lp A-I in postmenopausal women. *Atherosclerosis* 2002; **160**:495–501.

von Eckardstein A, Assmann G. Prevention of coronary heart disease by raising high-density lipoprotein cholesterol? *Curr Opin Lipidol* 2000;**11**:627-637.

Walldius G, Aastveit AH, Jungner I. Stroke mortality and the apoB/apoA-I ratio: results of the AMORIS prospective study. *J Intern Med* 2006; **259**: 259–66

Walldius G, Jungner I, Holme I, Aastveit AH, Kolar W, Steiner E. High apolipoprotein B, low polipoprotein A-I, and improvement in the prediction of fatal myocardial infarction AMORIS study): a prospective study. *Lancet* 2001; **358**:2026–33.

Walldius G, Jungner I. Apolipoprotein B and apolipoprotein A-I: risk indicators of coronary heart disease and targets for lipid-modifying therapy. *J Intern Med* 2004; **255**/2: 188–205.

Walldius G, Jungner I. Rationale for using apolipoprotein B and apolipoprotein A-I as indicators of cardiac risk and as targets for lipid-lowering therapy. *Eur Heart J* 2005; **26**: 210–2.

Wang, M.; Briggs, M. R. Chem. ReV. 2004; **104**, 119-137.

Weyer C, Bogardus C, Pratley RE. Metabolic characteristics of individuals with impaired fasting glucose and/ or impaired glucose tolerance. *Diabetes* 1999; **48**: 2197-2203.

WHO and ADA criteria for the diagnosis of diabetes mellitus in relation to body mass index. 2002; **26**:90-96.

Wing RR, Bunker CH, Kuller LH, Matthews KA: Insulin, body mass index, and cardiovascular risk factors in premenopausal women. *Arteriosclerosis* 1989; **9**:479-484.

Winocour PH, Durrington PN, Hunt L, Anderson DC, Cohen H: Effect of short-term improvements in glycaemic control on serum lipoprotcins in insuhn treated diabetes, in insulin treated diabetes, IN Crepaldi G, Teinzo A, Baggio G: *Diabetes, Obesity and Hyperlipidemia* 1985;681:269-270.

Winocour PH, Durrington PN, Ishola M, Anderson DC: Lipoprotein abnormalities in insulin-dependent diabetes meliitus. *Lancet* 1986; **1**:1176-1178.

Winocour PH, Ishola M, Durrington PN: Determinations of low density Iipoprotein cholesterol in insulin treated diabetes meliitus: A comparison of the Friedewald formula with direct measurement of very low density Iipoprotein cholesterol. *Clin Chim Acta* 1989; **179**:79-84.

Wynn V: Adverse effects of oral contraceptives, in Oliver MF, Vedin A, Wilhelmson C (eds): *Myocardial Infarction in Women*. Edinburgh, Churchill Livingstone, 1986, pp 103-116.

Zheng XL, Matsubara S, Diao C, Hollenberg MD, Wong NC: Activation of apolipoprotein AI gene expression by protein kinase A and kinase C through transcription factor, Sp1. *J Biol Chem* 2000; **275**:31747–31754.

Zimmet PZ. Diabetes epidemiology as a tool to trigger diabetes research and care. *Diabetologia* 1999; **42**: 499-518.

Zunic G, Jelic-Ivanovic Z, Spasic S,Stojiljkovik A, Majkic-Singh N. Reference value for Apolipoproteins A-I and B in Healthy Subjects, by age. *Clin Chem* 1992;38:566-569.

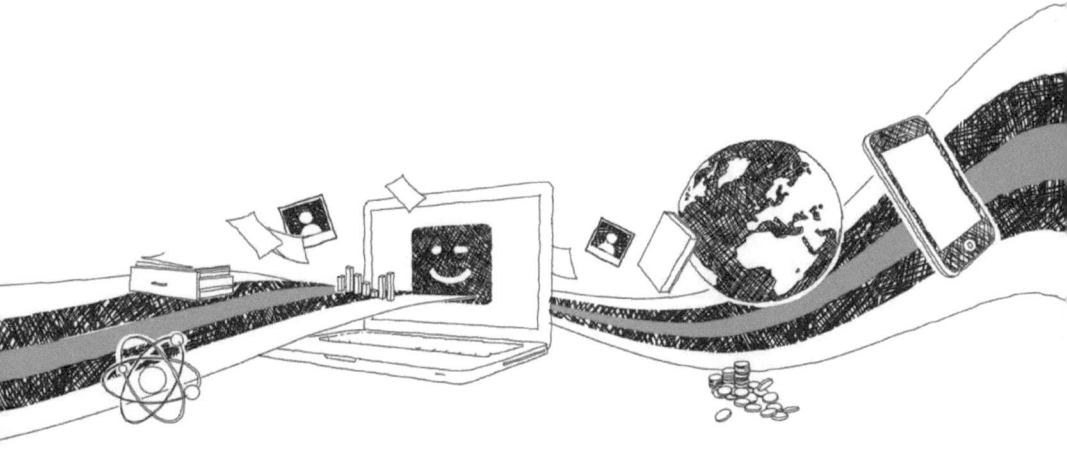
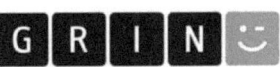